Millions of Women
Discover Susan Nethero's Bra Talk

"I was so desperate I wanted breast reduction surgery," says Ana, an actress, singer, and dancer. "I was miserable in my body and in my heart. My mom phoned me after seeing you on television and told me to go to your store. Once I got there, it seemed to take only thirty glorious seconds to find bras that reduced my breast size by at least one cup. Thank you so much for making me happy and healthy again."

"Before you fitted me properly in the right bra, I thought I was deformed or something." — says Christina

"I finally feel like a normal person." — Cheryl

"Thank you for giving me my body back!" — Jennifer

"You changed my life!" — Sarah

Now *you*, too, can benefit from the same **Bra Talk** tips, advice, facts, and myths Susan Nethero has shared with the devoted customers of her INTIMACY lingerie shops and with audiences across the country.

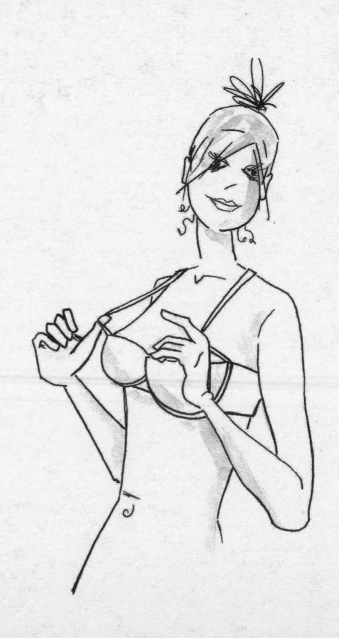

BraTalk

BraTalk

myths and facts

transform your life with the right bra fit

Susan Nethero

nationally known bra-fitting expert

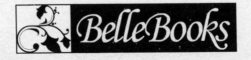

Smyrna, Georgia

BelleBooks

ISBN number 0-9768760-0-0

Bra Talk

Copyright 2005 by Susan Nethero

Printed and bound in the United States.

Published by

BelleBooks

P.O. Box 67

Smyrna, GA 30081

www.bellebooks.com

10 9 8 7 6 5 4 3 2 1

Cover and interior design by John Cole

Illustrations by Robbi Dare

Author photograph by Lizzy Sullivan

Dedication

To my Intimacy fitters and management staff, who have shown through their years of buying, client relations and fit/style service that in satisfying each and every client we've brought forth the good for all other women to see.

To my daughters — please know — when you are passionate to learn all there is to know about the work you love, then you can endure the challenges and obstacles you face along the way. Staying the course and being consistent in your dedication brings forth great rewards.

To my husband, who listened, trusted and inspired me with his unconditional support over many years and who gave me the freedom to pursue my professional life because he understood my personal need for achievement and my passion to create life-changing experiences for women.

To our business friends and customers, who encouraged us to tell our story and have remained close by our sides for many years.

To Rena, always a faithful friend to our family, for her love, spiritual insights, and infinite wisdom, which inspires each one of us to live and fulfill our potential.

To Toni, our heavenly fitting angel, uplifting all of us with her passion. We dearly miss you.

Susan

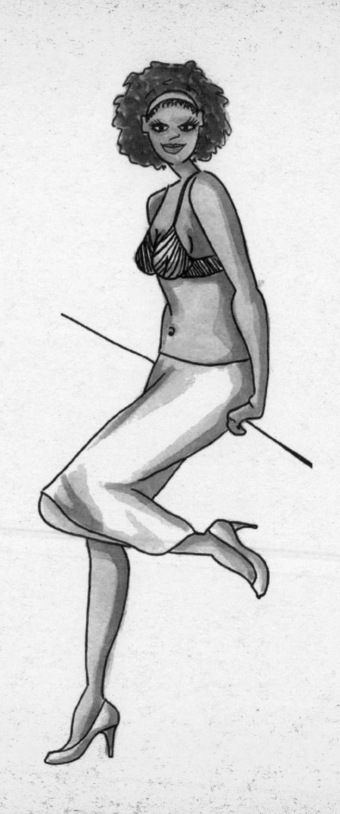

Your Bra Talk Resource Guide

"Jiggle, wiggle, bounce, ouch! I love my breasts, but I hate my bra. Help!"

Many women feel powerless to change the way their breasts look and feel. Conventional beauty and makeover programs rarely address the subject of picking the right bra for each woman's unique needs. So we struggle onward, hoping to find new ways to enhance our figures. For most of us, there's high emotion and drama in the shape and appearance of our breasts.

Research shows that 85% of all women — over 90 million women in the United States, alone! — are wearing the wrong-sized bra. As a result, most women suffer in their look, style and comfort. Thanks to today's clinging fashions, it really shows! Just take a quick survey of your friends, family and co-workers — and take a look at yourself in the mirror. Pretend you're a fashion cop on the beat. Get out your ticket book and record the number of obvious bra violations.

It's a small wonder our bouncing bust lines don't stop traffic. They're truly out of control!

How can one of the most private articles of clothing be so challenging to select? Why are so few women happy about their foundations? Sadly, few women feel their bras enhance their figures or make them feel beautiful.

That's why I'm passionate about helping women transform their appearance and, by extension, their self-confidence. As a professional bra fitter I've witnessed some amazing success stories over the years.

I strive to share the following message via my shops, my radio and TV appearances and in magazine articles:

There's no such thing as one perfect bra for all women!

Thus, I've written *Bra Talk* to help you overcome the myths, avoid the fashion *faux pas*, get the facts about bra fit and learn how you can find your own comfort, shape and beauty. Let's talk bras!

— Susan Nethero

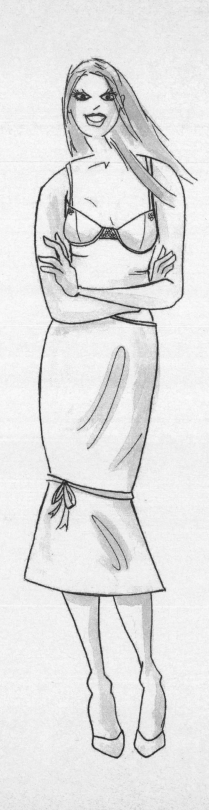

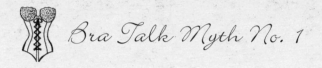

Bra Talk Myth No. 1

No matter our age or condition, our breasts don't change very much.

"I haven't switched my bra style since high school. Why should I?"

Here's the fact: The average woman's breasts change size and shape six times in her life. Some of the reasons?

- Weight loss or gain
- Increase or decrease in exercise
- Use of birth control pills or hormone replacement therapy
- Pregnancy and nursing
- Changes in diet/nutrition
- Breast implants

Most women don't realize how much they're affected by those factors. It's thought-provoking to understand how often our bodies change for reasons we can't control. Yet we're told we *have* to control our shapes and sizes, not to mention our *lives*. Every day, we struggle to diet and exercise to maintain or regain a trim and youthful body. Through puberty, childbirth and menopause, we watch our bodies evolve despite our best efforts. However, the many other life changes a woman experiences also stress her body and bust size. Most women will experience one or more changes in her breasts every five years of her life.

> A staggering 55% of all women report one or more breast changes during the past year.

Weight Changes

Weight loss or gain can alter your bra size and your requirements for good support. The elasticity of your breast tissue may be reduced, causing loss of firmness — especially if your weight loss or gain is greater than ten percent of your body weight.

Exercise

Exercising is great, but it doesn't build up your breasts.

Why not? Because when we increase or decrease our exercise level, we change our body fat. A decline in body fat reduces a woman's bra size and, in some cases, the firmness of her breasts. Breast tissue is not a muscle.

Yes, it's true that younger women can use exercise to tighten the pectoral muscles that lie behind the breast tissue, thus improving the uplift of the entire breast. But exercise can also stress the breast and cause loss of firmness — despite the positive benefits of exercise for fitness and well-being.

No matter your age, always wear a good bra when you exercise. A sports bra will greatly improve the support and firmness that is beneficial for breast health and will reduce breast injury from excessive or intense sports.

Birth Control Pills and Hormone Therapy

Birth control pills and hormone replacement therapy often cause women to retain water and significantly affect their hormone levels. Usually, this increases a woman's breast size one cup size. Cortisone-based medications can also influence fluid retention and often increase a woman's breast size.

Pregnancy and Nursing

Pregnancy and/or nursing places demand on the breast tissue and skin resilience. Most women lose firmness due to increases of at least 1-2 cup sizes. The constant fill-up and release of milk during lactation stresses the breast. For the expectant mom, it would be advisable to buy nursing bras with extra room in the cup depth. Consider a soft-cup bra without an underwire, as the milk ducts are located at the root of the breast.

Changes in Diet

Changes in diet may affect the percentages of body fat, fluids or protein your body needs to metabolize and nourish the breast tissue. Radical changes in diet can also result in hormone imbalance and loss of hair. Always remember — what's bad for your body is generally bad for your breasts, too.

Breast Implants

Even if you've got implants, your breasts require the same support as any other woman's. Skin elasticity and resilience is highly individual and often influenced more by genetic history than how the implant is placed (either under or over the pectoral muscle.)

> **Bra Talk Tip:** Your bra size will vary depending on the style of bra. Designers have tried to standardize bra sizes, but differences still exist. Don't ever buy a bra without trying it on, first! You'll discover that seamed cups have more depth and distribute cup volume better, so they feel more comfortable. You may wear a smaller cup size in a seamed bra. On the other hand, you'll almost always need to go up a cup size if you switch to a seamless bra. Seamless cups are generally rigid and have less flexibility. Manufacturers add comfort by incorporating greater stretch in the back.

Dear Bra Talk: In sixth grade, when all of the girls in my class started developing, the most popular question asked by boys was, "Are those bug bites?"

Bra Talk Tours Your Collection Of Misfit Bras, Rejected Bras, And Bad Bargain Bras

Admit it. Somewhere in the darkest recesses of your lingerie drawer lurk *The Zombie Bras Of Doom*. Otherwise known as, "Bras I Wish I Hadn't Bought."

Just look through your drawer and count the number of bras you've pushed to the back in favor of your comfy favorites. All of us have done it — bought a bra but then decided after a few wearings that we want to scream from the pain or discomfort. If you've ever felt guilty over those regretable purchases or frustrated because you wasted your money on an unwearable bra, then you're not alone. Look at this statistic:

It's estimated that half of all purchased bras end up languishing in lingerie drawers. That's right. One out of every two bras is a Zombie Bra of Doom. It's a wonder when you find a bra that's right for you!

That's why I contend that a professionally fitted bra actually *saves* you money. No more dollars wasted on Zombies! Instead, invest in good, wearable bras, and ultimately your satisfaction and wardrobe will increase.

You can't hold up a D cup with a five-dollar bra. Concentrate on quality and proper fit, and your investment will be worthwhile.

Bra Talk Tip: You need a minimum of three good bras: One to wear, one in the wash, and one on stand-by, in the lingerie drawer. Ultimately, you should add another couple of bras to your collection, building to a wardrobe of seven-to-ten well-fitting bras that you really, truly love and wear regularly. Not a Zombie Bra in sight!

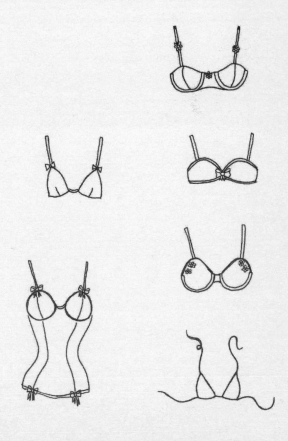

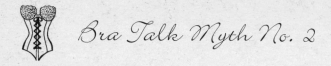 *Bra Talk Myth No. 2*

Bras aren't supposed to be comfortable.

> "I find myself racing to my car at the end of the day so I can unsnap my binding bra!"

You've done it in the office restroom.

You've done it in the car.

You may even have done it outside your mother-in-law's front door!

You *know* what I'm talking about. Freeing the hostages. Letting the puppies out of their pen. Springing the twins from the booby hatch.

Taking off your painful, ill-fitting bra.

You race home from work — maybe even sneak your bra off in the car! Women tell me they rip off their uncomfortable bras in the *weirdest* places — just to feel that glorious *ahhhhh* of relief.

Are bras *supposed* to hurt? No!

So why do we think it's acceptable for underwires to cause discomfort and irritation to our breasts? Women have been told by the media and medical community that underwires are unhealthy. Some experts say, "Wear a soft cup, instead!"

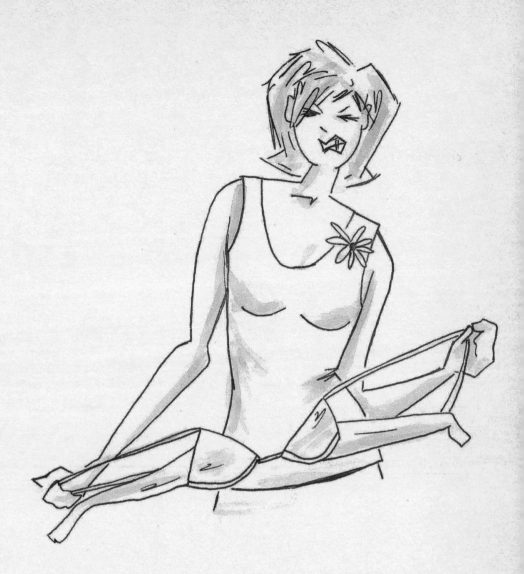

Not true!

We've also been led to believe it's normal for our bras to shift on our bodies during the day. We accept the annoyance of constantly adjusting our shoulder or back band. Again, not necessary!

And on top of it all, we think we have no choice but to give into that dreaded affliction known as "bulging back fat." No way!

Despite endless fashion articles about bra fit, cup sizing and fashion styles, many women simply have come to believe, "Bras are not supposed to be comfortable." We seem to think we're to blame for the poor fit. I suspect a lot of us put up with ill-fitting bras because we're a little embarrassed to ask for professional help. We may fear the loss of privacy with a professional bra fitting. Will be it be humiliating and uncomfortable?

Let me set the record straight: It may seem impossible to find a great bra — but it's not rocket science! It doesn't require an engineering degree, a tape measure and a chart on bra-fitting mathematics to deduce your cup size before you go shopping.

Everyone should experience the dramatic benefit of a personalized bra fitting — it's life changing, and it's fun!

So don't hesitate. Get help, don't live with discomfort, get the right fit!

Bra Talk **From The Heart**

- *Stephani's Story* -

Dear Susan,

I am sixteen years old. I recently was in the school musical, starring in a lead role in one of my all-time favorite plays. Rehearsals were fun and so was singing my favorite songs with all my friends. It was all fun and games until dress rehearsal came along.

My costume included a tight-fitting top. The same tight, '*sexy*' top that all the other girls in the cast were excited about because it made them look like they had more than just 'mosquito bites' on their chests. But that top made *me* look stupid! It made my humongous water balloons look more saggy than usual. It turned me into a chubby little girl.

"That was my defining moment."

I was not going to let my great time be ruined by saggy breasts and a terrible costume. I was not going to let the other girls look better than me. And I was definitely ready to stop my breasts from 'coming out all over the place,' as my friends often chastised me about.

It had always been a running joke: Stephanie, the girl with the huge boobs. I was ready to face the facts and get a new bra that actually fit.

My mom and I headed to one of those well-known lingerie stores that carries sexy stuff. I wanted all the fun, thrilling lingerie that all girls, me included, look up to as sexy and scandalous. We went to the back of the shop and found a woman with a tape measure around her neck, ready to answer the one treacherous question this sixteen-year-old girl was about to confront her with: "What size am I?"

The answer came soon. Oh, it came.

She measured my width, and she measured my cup. It turned out I fit into a triple D! This famous store, this mature, sexy store, didn't have *anything* that fit me.

As my mother and I left, I looked back at the unattainable lingerie. No matter how much I dieted or exercised, no matter how self-assured I became, I'd never be allowed to wear those garments. Simply because this sixteen-year-old girl was too big to be sexy.

Or so I thought.

"I was in heaven."

About a week later, my mom and I heard about *Intimacy*. After the huge emotional ordeal at the other store, I wasn't particularly excited to go to yet another shop that did not carry anything in my bust size.

I was so wrong! At *Intimacy*, a consultant fit me in a G cup. She gave me halter tops, sexy bras, tank tops, bathing suits, and strapless bras galore. I was in heaven. I began to cry. I was finally in a store that had seen people like me, before.

I bought a bra that looked great with my costume, and with my everyday clothes. I got clothes that looked great on my body and made me *feel* great. Thank you for making this sixteen-year-old girl feel at home, with people who finally cared.

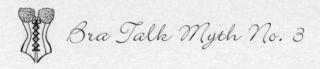

A loose-fitting bra is the most comfortable.

"It's almost like going braless, isn't it?"

We live in America, the land of *big* ideas and the home of the " Bigger is Better" life philosophy. It's part of our culture and our most basic beliefs. We associate comfort and looseness with freedom, so most women, when they notice their clothing is a bit snug, will go up a size to solve the problem. Since we women tend to feel bad about our bodies, we often blame ourselves for fit issues. But even if you're a supermodel (tall and lean), you'll find some part of your figure unacceptable to your self image or the shape you wish you had. But wearing a bra that fits like a baggy bandeau only makes the problem worse.

Contrary to popular opinion, the most comfortable bra is the one that fits firmly. Our bras work 14-16 hours a day to lift the bust and hold the body. With active lifestyles, we need performance from our bras! Constantly readjusting a loose, baggy bra is irritating to you and your body. Not to mention, embarrassing!

A firm-fitting bra should give you a feeling of security — like being held and supported. Once you put on your bra, you shouldn't have to think about it again. It doesn't shift. It supports and evenly distributes the weight of the breasts and results in increased comfort, even after the longest day. It lifts the breasts as if it's a natural part of your body.

Bra Talk Fitting Tip: The perfect bra should fit snugly to your body even with the back band in its loosest hook position. It may feel different or "odd" when you go from a 38 to a 34, but you'll find the bra relaxes after one or two wearings, and soon you won't be conscious it's even on your body. Remember: If it's saggy in the loosest hook position when it's brand new, it'll be even worse later on.

You want to be able to tighten the bra as it relaxes with wear and the warmth of your body. You want it to retain the support it gives you when it's new.

In this sense, buying a bra is like buying shoes: If you buy shoes that are too loose to begin with, in no time at all you'll be clomping around in a pair of shoes that are too big for you. A bra is very similar.

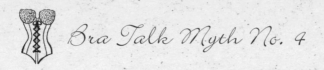

Minimizer bras are the best hope for making large breasts look smaller.

"A bra's supposed to act like a girdle for big boobs, right?"

Women who want to make their busts look small often buy "minimizer" bras. Minimizers can be found everywhere in the U.S. market, and are available from many major bra makers. I don't like them at all. I think they deceive large-breasted women who really want to improve their figures, not bind their chests. Why?

Minimizers compress the breast tissue over the entire chest cavity, spreading additional volume under the arm, and up and down the chest. But all that additional volume on the body tends to make a woman's upper body look *thick* by increasing the surface area of the breast on her torso.

Bad idea.

A full-busted woman needs all the torso length she can get in order to look well proportioned. Women who wear minimizer bras look as if they've padded their waistlines.

So what's the solution? Don't smash your large breasts flat. Lift them higher. If a woman wants to looks smaller busted, she should raise her breasts and narrow the width of the bust line so her breasts aren't wider than her body frame.

The combination of those two techniques will give her full breasts extra lift, make her torso look longer, and slim her upper body frame. When I fit full-busted women with the right bra, they feel as if they've lost ten pounds, and their clothes fit better.

No more saggy bust lines. Now their breasts look full and natural. Big-breasted gals should celebrate their curves. Vavoom!

Bra Talk Fact: It's important for women to know that compressing breast tissue is unhealthy for their breasts. It causes loss of firmness and generally doesn't support the bust. Most minimizer bras don't have sufficient cup depth to support the breasts or protect the tissue beneath the arms from continuous bumping with any movement. Many women wearing minimizers also complain that the underwires ride up when they lift their arms. Ouch! That hurts!

Dear Bra Talk: My sister's boyfriend told me I will never drown, because I have built-in flotation devices.

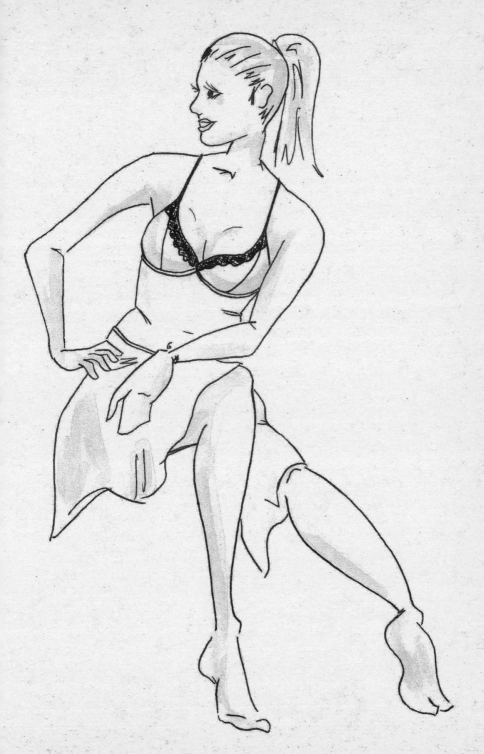

17

Bra Talk About Bra Wear And Care

Don't give your bra a premature death.

Sound a bit crazy? The truth is, you can greatly extend the life of your bra with the right care.

Remember, a bra is a high-tech product of fashion engineering. You need to pamper its modern materials. Those soft, buttery, beautiful, microfibers will lose their elasticity if you abuse them with rough wear and harsh detergents.

If your bra had a motto, it would be: *Wear me, but don't wear me out!*

Rotate your bras. Give them days off. In general, you should wear a bra only *two* times before washing it — and I don't mean two days in a row. Rest your bra between wearings. I'm serious. Your bra relaxes with the warmth of your body. If you wear the same bra constantly, it will lose its firmness.

A clean bra is a contented bra.

When you wash your bra, you should always use cool water. Cool water shocks the elastic, helping the bra retain its stretch and shape. Choose a delicate soap — no chlorinating agents, please! Soaps I recommend:

- Forever New (designed specifically for lingerie)
- Deft
- Ivory Snow

Woolite, while known as a great specialty soap, is designed for cleaning natural fibers — wool — and thus I don't recommend it for the synthetic fibers, such as Lycra, used by lingerie manufacturers.

If you're traveling and you don't have any lingerie soap handy, use your shampoo.

Whatever you do, don't wash your bra in hot water. Hot water will shrink the cotton felt that covers your underwires, and the wires may pop out.

My bras have a cushy life. What next?

It's always best to wash them by hand. If you *must* put your bras in a washing machine, at least protect them in a net lingerie bag. Fasten the back band securely, and use the delicate cycle. Do *not* put your bras in the dryer! The temperatures are too hot. The average dryer actually *cooks* any residual soap left in the bra's fibers. That causes loss of firmness, which cannot be regained. Instead, dry your bras the way Mother Nature intended: slowly, in open air.

Pamper your bras, and they'll pamper *you* with years of quality service.

> **Bra Talk Tip:** Don't try to fix falling shoulder straps by shortening them. Instead, tighten your back band and make sure it's pulled down properly.

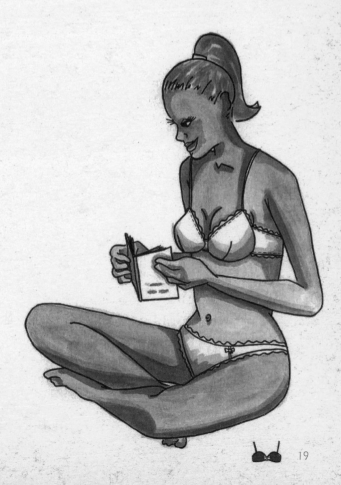

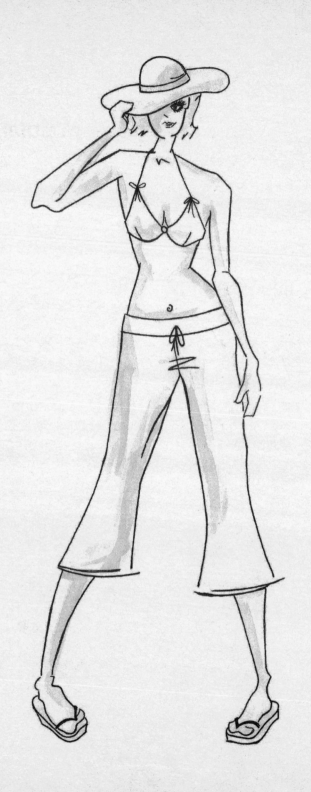

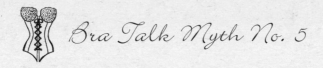

If a bra's trendy and popular, surely it's perfect for me, too.

"You mean I shouldn't choose a bra just because it looks good on Paris Hilton?"

Sometimes it seems everyone falls in love with the bra of the moment. Perhaps they've seen it in a fashion magazine or heard it endorsed by a popular television personality. Or maybe a friend has gushed about her new push-up bra or invisible latex straps. Some new bras are marketed as fashion statements, and others for a special performance feature.

We love to catch a trend. Newness sells! We want to wear the latest, greatest, *perfect* bra! Don't be fooled: Every new bra is always touted as the "perfect" bra when it's launched on the market.

But perfection doesn't come from a one-style-fits-all bra. It comes from a proper fit, with styling that compliments *your* individual figure and bust size. A bra is perfect when it gives a woman's breasts the right definition, shape and beauty, whether she's a petite *A* cup or a full *DD*. So what's good for you may be uniquely different from your best friend. And the latest fashion trend may be a fatal fashion mistake for *you*.

Bra Talk Tip: Professional bra fitters will evaluate styles that will compliment your figure. If you've lost firmness, she'll select shaping and lightly lined contour cups or rigid cup styles that really support and give you the best proportionate shape. With a perfect fit, you'll feel like a whole new woman!

Bra Talk **From the Heart**

- Sarah's Story -

Dear Susan,

I have been small-busted all my life. Bra shopping has never been easy for me. I always assumed I was an A cup. However, I could never find a bra that fit me well. Every chance I could, I would try on as many A cup bras as I could find. As we all know, that size cup is not very prevalent in many mainstream bra stores or department stores, so I never found too many.

"I would usually end up in tears."

The hunt was quite frustrating, and I would usually end up in tears. I found myself wearing my old bras and sports bras. Those were the only bras that would fit me comfortably.

One day at lunch, a fellow small-busted co-worker and I were discussing how tough it is for us to find bras that fit. She suggested I go to *Intimacy* and get fitted. I was in the store within a week!

A sales associate came into the dressing room and asked me about my bra history. I told her that 32A was too small and 34A was too big. What to do? She told me I must be a 32B or bigger. I thought 'bigger. . .is she *kidding* me?'

I have such a tiny chest there is no way I could be in a bigger cup size than A.

The clerk came back with several bras, and I began trying on some cute 32B styles. Some fit but some were snug, so she then had me try on some 32C bras. Lo and behold, they fit! I *never* would have *ever* thought to try on 32C, yet this clerk could tell just by looking at me and hearing my frustrations that 32B or 32C would be a perfect fit.

I was thrilled!

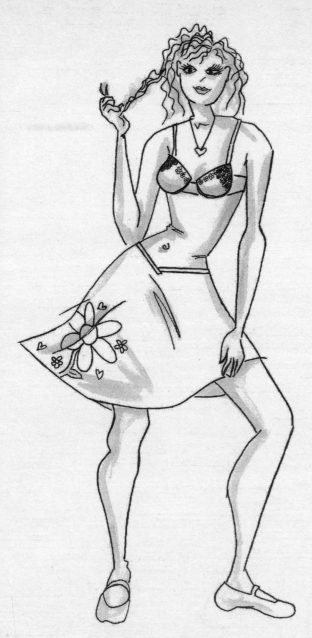

I ended up buying three bras that day. When I met back with my friends, I began to cry with excitement. All the frustrations and heartaches I had experienced over years of bra shopping were extinguished in a thirty-minute visit to a specialist.

My experience was life-changing. Plus, my husband was thrilled to find out he had married a woman who wears a C cup!

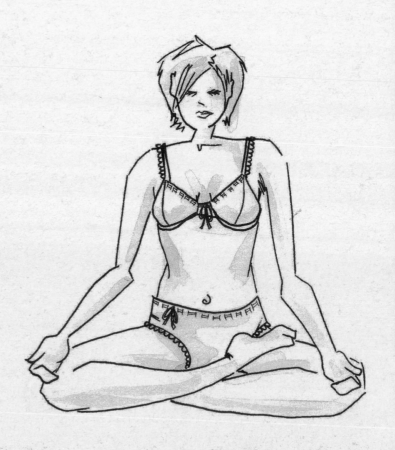

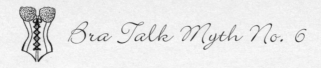

Cup sizes aren't that important to a good fit.

"What's the deal about cup sizing? I'm a B cup. Aren't all B cups the same size? And are U.S. sizes different from European?"

It seems so easy to pick a cup size. We're all used to grading systems. It's just like school, isn't it? In school, if you score between 90 and 100 on a test, you get an A. If you score between 80 and 89, you earn a B. Simple. Just measure yourself.

But it's trickier with bra sizing. I estimate that only one in five women understand the differences in bra cups. So if the next few facts come as a surprise to you, you're not alone!

> **Bra Talk Fact:** Bra cup sizes are proportionate to the body frame. That's right, cups get progressively larger as the bra's back band gets larger. In other words, a 36B cup is two cup sizes deeper than a 32B. Every time you go up a back size the cup gets one size larger!

Bra designers created that sizing standard decades ago, based on the idea that as a woman's body gets larger her bra cups should become fuller. Sounds reasonable, but there's more to it. With each increase in back length, the cups get one-inch deeper in volume, but also, they move farther apart! You heard right. Manufacturers increase the bra's centerpiece (that small piece of material between the cups) to adjust for a larger-frame woman.

Clients tell me all the time: "I carry wide," meaning their breasts are not "centered." But in fact, that's rare. Most of the time, a woman doesn't realize she's wearing a bra made for someone with a larger frame — so, *of course*, she looks like her breasts are too far apart. They're heading east and west instead of straight ahead!

> **Bra Talk Tip:** If your bra feels snug or uncomfortable, don't automatically assume all you need is a longer band. Your problem is most likely the cup size, instead.

Many women still buy the same cup size even when their band length has increased. I'll hear a client say, "Oh, I've always been a C cup." But when I ask her if her band size has changed she tells me she's gone from a 34 to a 38 (that's an increase of two cup sizes!) Clearly, she doesn't realize that her cups have become proportionately larger.

Changes in a woman's cup size happen over a number of years. Maybe she's not as firm as she used to be. Now her breasts don't quite fill the cups, or her sloping tissue falls to the bottoms of the cups, and she can't understand why she's lost volume. She sees a gap between the upper part of the bra cups and her breasts. She doesn't realize she can fix those problems by going down one cup size.

Are You An Espresso Or A Grandé Latté?

The Bra Talk Guide To Cup Sizes

The Espresso

If you're an A cup, you need more fullness to create your ideal proportions. Try a padded demi-bra (a half-cup bra,) or a lightly lined contour-shaping bra. If you fall in love with a sheer cup bra, add silicone gel inserts.

The Cappuccino

You B cup women can add fullness, too! Try a plunging demi-cup bra or a contour bra that accentuates the definition of your breast shape. Focus on the size of the bra and on filling the cup volume.

The Diner Classic

Congratulations! You're a C cup, and that puts you in the majority. You'll find most bras are designed for your size. You can enjoy a sheer-cup bra or a seamless, molded cup because you have sufficient volume to create a natural shape. Look for bras with vertical cup seams to maximize your fullness.

The Grandé Latté

As a D cup woman, you have ample fullness. You're able to wear most bra styles with ease and look your best. You can wear a sheer cup or a seamless, molded bra and fill the cup depth. A diagonally seamed bra will usually give you a little more support and will also give you maximum slimness. Take advantage of your beautiful cleavage!

The Grandé Latté With Extra Milk

If you wear a DD or larger cup size, look for additional levels of support in your bras. Select styles that give you structure and narrow the width of your bust line so that it's well within your body frame. A seamless bra that is rigid or double-lined will give you natural fullness and reduce the appearance of sloped or sagging breasts. A seamed bra will generally make you look narrower (meaning slimmer!) because the depth of the cup is greater. A seamed, multi-sectioned cup helps direct your breasts forward, instead of letting them splay to the sides.

Don't worry about a fuller bust – when your bust is full it makes your hips look narrower! Accentuate your "Barbie-like" proportions!

"So, what cup size am I, really, and how the heck do I figure it out?"

Start by determining your back width — that is, your circumference — with this handy, quick guide.

Blouse Size	0-2	4-6	8-10	12-14	16-18	1x	2x
Bra Band Size	30	32	34	36	38	40	42

So, let's suppose you wear a size 8 blouse. Then the bra size most appropriate for you would be a 34. The following chart shows the solid lines between cup sizes which are exactly the same cup depth. For example, a 36B is equivalent in cup volume to a 34C or a 32D. Begin by pinpointing what size bra you currently wear. Next, identify your approximate blouse size at the bottom of the chart. Follow the solid line down or up the chart from your current bra size to your correct blouse size.

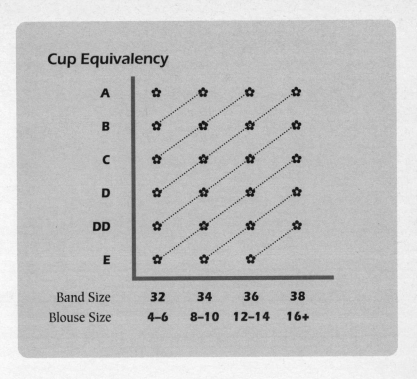

Cup Equivalency

	32	34	36	38
A	✿	✿	✿	✿
B	✿	✿	✿	✿
C	✿	✿	✿	✿
D	✿	✿	✿	✿
DD	✿	✿	✿	✿
E	✿	✿	✿	

Band Size	32	34	36	38
Blouse Size	4–6	8–10	12–14	16+

Balancing the two sizes can seem confusing, I know. See a professional fitter to get expert advice. It's worth the visit!

Bra Talk Tip: Are you full figured? Do you have a thick midriff, so sometimes your bra's back band feels too tight? Consider going up one cup size rather than buying a bigger back band. Why? When your cups are too small the tension tugs on your back band, making it feel tighter. So buy a bigger cup size and you'll take the pressure off the band. You should feel a big improvement. To make sure you're buying a comfortably sized back band, sit down when you try on a new bra. Your rib cage will expand a little, so you get a truer fit and a "real life" test.

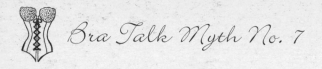

Bra Talk Myth No. 7

When it comes to size, close enough is good enough.

"My size is hard to find. Sales clerks insist I can wear a different one. What gives?"

Many stores will recommend a *conversion* size to you if they don't stock your true size. But when a sales clerk offers you a substitute, will that bra fit you properly? I doubt it. Yes, the conversion size will have the same cup depth as the size you requested. However, the back band will be at least one size too large!

This is *not* a good alternative! The bra will shift on your body and stretch with wear. When a bra is too big around, you lose support and lift within a few wearings.

Bra manufacturers still don't give women a good selection of bras in every size range. Many U.S. bra makers only want to produce the most popular sizes, the ones they can manufacture with greatest efficiency at the lowest cost.

The biggest retail stores tend to stock only about a dozen key sizes. Frankly, that's a disservice to all of us. But take heart: If your bra size falls outside the average B or C cup, you may find your perfect size in a European brand. Many U.S. department stores assume that only full-figured gals have fuller busts! That's not true. Most specialized bra shops, including my own, carry special sizes and European brands. Did you know there are over *seventy-five sizes* from which to choose?

Bra Talk Tip: For a list of specialty bra-fitting shops near your home, see the nationwide store locator at www.myintimacy.com. You'll find over 100 specialty stores in thirty-two states! And we're always adding new stores to the list.

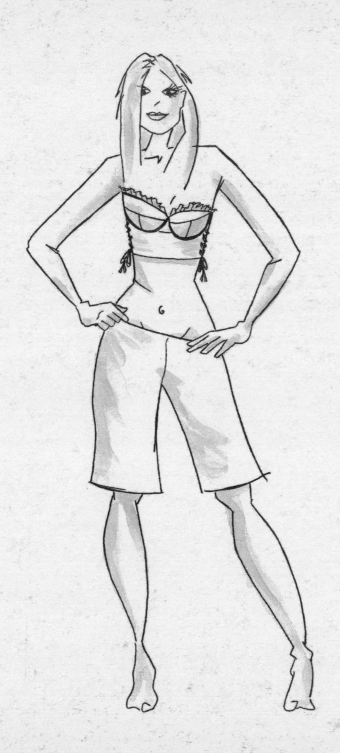

Bra Talk Tip: If you want to add some temporary *vavoom!* to perk up a low-cut dress or slinky top, switch to a padded bra. A good one can make you look at least a half-cup size bigger. Also tighten up the bra's shoulder straps an inch or so.

Dear Bra Talk: I've always been flat-chested, and my younger sister has bigger breasts than I do. In elementary school, my friend, Warren, used to tell me I should rub onions and garlic on my breasts to make them grow. I refused. When my sister's breasts grew, Warren insisted I should have taken his advice.

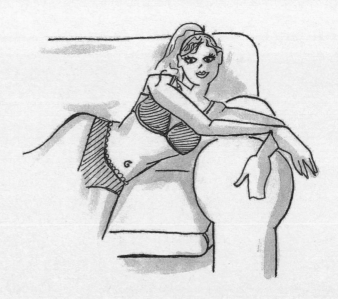

The Good, The Bad and The Droopy
Bra Talk Breast Facts

Here comes the science!

Your breasts are composed of fat, milk glands, rubbery fibers, blood vessels, and skin. They have no muscle or other tissue that can be exercised or developed.

So here's the bad news: Eventually, your boobs will sag. It's just a fact of nature and gravity.

As you age, your breasts lose firmness and begin to slope. Stretch marks may appear. Your upper breasts lose their plump, youthful volume.

Imagine the weight of your breasts pulling on your neck, shoulders, and chest wall. Glue a penny to the end of a rubber band and suspend it from your window sill. In six months the rubber band won't lengthen much. But after a year or two — or twenty-five or fifty — you'd see a major difference in the elasticity.

Your breasts are made up of hundreds of "rubber bands."

Without the proper bra support, gravity takes hold and your breasts begin to slide down your chest. As horrible as it sounds, without proper support your breast tissue can actually *detach* from your chest wall. When this occurs, blood flow to the breasts is interrupted and the breast tissue is bumped and battered with every move.

The breast tissue will re-attach lower on your chest once it's stable, and blood flow will be restored, but the damage is done! Only expensive plastic surgery can restore breasts that have headed south to retire.

> **Bra Talk Tip:** Sing along, now: Do your breasts hang low, do they wobble to and fro, can you tie 'em in a knot, can you tie 'em in a bow . . .Girlfriend, you need lift and shape. Buy bras with contour cups or *heat-seamed* cups that will get you back on top of your game! Just make sure the bra's centerpiece doesn't plunge too low, or you may fall out!

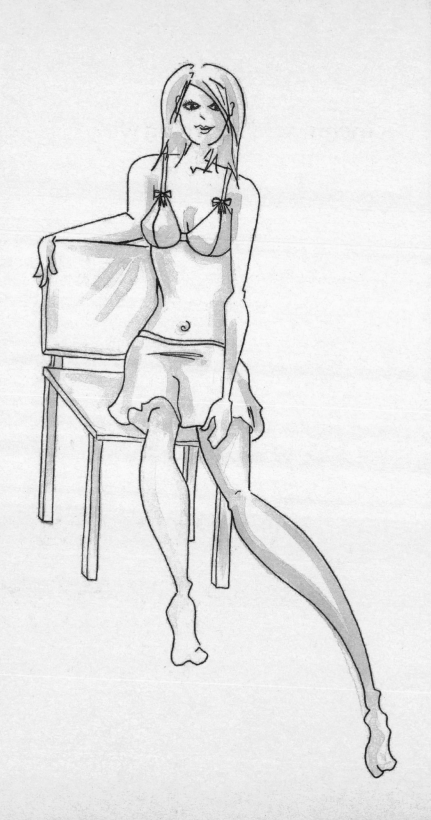

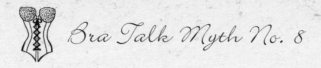 *Bra Talk Myth No. 8*

There's nothing wrong with the bras, it's your body's fault.

> "I have embarrassing shape issues.
> That's why bras never fit me right."

Women tell me their fitting problems as if they're confessing a crime. Let me be very clear about this: Your body is fine. It's the bra that needs to serve hard time, not you.

Research has shown that all women suffer the same general problems with their bras, regardless of differences in size and shape. Our tendency to blame ourselves for fashion faux pas is all too common! But it's unfair and untrue, and I refuse to allow women to suffer the blame. Bra wearers of the world, unite!

The most amazing transformation happens when a woman finally sees how great she can look in the right bra. Her confidence and self-esteem improve instantly. The *uplifting* experience isn't just physical, it's emotional.

The truth is, most women don't realize how much difference a well-fitted bra can make until they actually see the results. Every woman has beautiful features that can and should be highlighted! Whether you're petite or full busted — you deserve to experience the comfort, definition and dramatic effects of a perfect bra fitting.

So don't blame your body for something that's your bra's fault! How can you be comfortable with your body if you're not comfortable with your bra? Indulge yourself! The right bra gives your entire body a facelift!

Bra Talk Tips: What you can expect from a professional bra fitter.

- ⚇ She'll educate you about your correct size.
- ⚇ She'll show you which styles are good for your body type and shape.
- ⚇ She'll recommend specific bras designed for your individual lifestyle.
- ⚇ She'll teach you how to take care of your bra so it stays in great condition.

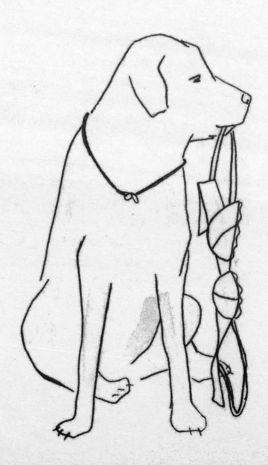

Bra Talk **From The Heart**

- Rebecca's Story -

Dear Susan,

My daughter and I are both large-busted. We went to a bra fitting for her sake. She's young and none of her clothes fit properly. She was always having to buy 'old lady bras.' Plus my husband had been urging *me* to find bras that really fit.

So when my daughter came home for spring break, I kidnapped her! I didn't tell her where we were going, or she never would have come. We went to your store for a fitting. My intent was to get a bra for myself, but also buy my daughter several. When she realized where I was taking her, my daughter was *not* happy with me at all.

We walked in, and a consultant took us to be fitted. She knew it was an uncomfortable situation for my daughter, and really catered to her youthful tastes. She explained why our old bras didn't fit, then she explained why lace bras are more supportive for women our size. My daughter and I tried on some bras and could see the difference right away.

Now my shoulders don't hurt at the end of the day. My posture has improved, as well. I feel better about the way I look. I can wear beautiful bras — and they don't have a back on them the width of a double-wide trailer! I stand taller and with a little more confidence. My breasts and my waist no longer join together. I have a torso now!

What I really love is seeing my daughter being able to wear really cute and pretty bras that she was never able to wear, before. Thank you!

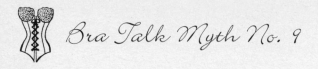

It's normal for a bra to cause neck, back and shoulder pain.

"Do I have to use shoulder pads?
I'm starting to look like a football player!"

Bench those bulky strap pads. If you're in pain, it may be because your straps are doing too much support duty. The end result of over-loaded shoulder straps is muscle tension, muscle fatigue, and loss of blood flow to the arms. Which is why observant doctors and chiropractors often recommend that women suffering from those ailments try a new bra. Ask your doctor for advice, absolutely!

> **Bra Talk Tip:** Many of our major arteries are located in the base of our lower necks and across our shoulders. Excessive pressure on those arteries can *easily* create numbness in your arms and fingers and an aching sensation in your neck. Not to mention permanent grooves in our shoulders! But a well-fitted underwire bra will take up to *90 percent* of your breasts' weight off the shoulder straps! And a good-fitting bra doesn't need wide straps to support you! You can feel fashionable and achieve good lift without looking as if you're wearing industrial-strength bras.

Every woman's body is a unique work of art. A woman endures, overcomes, and even *celebrates* a daunting array of transitions through out her life — transitions that put her mind and body to the test. So I say this: If changing your bra doesn't solve your pain problem, you may want to talk to your doctor about breast reduction.

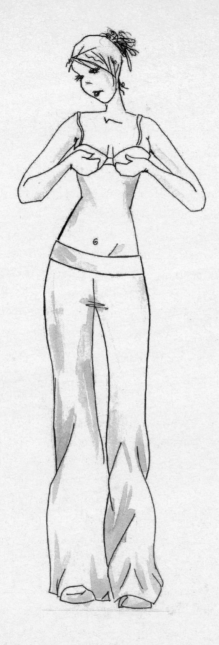

Even the best, most professionally fitted bra won't resolve body-image issues for some women who feel especially defeated by their breast size. In my experience, women who've had a breast reduction feel the rewards are well worth the risks.

Fashion Versus Function
Some Uplifting Bra Talk Facts

"Is there really much difference in quality between a 'fashion bra' I buy for fun and a hardworking bra I intend to wear every day?"

You bet there's a difference! A quality bra may contain as many as *forty* pieces and take 24-30 months from design inception to finished product. A lower-quality bra may take only 12-15 months to design and manufacture (due to fewer grading/wear tests and revision cycles) and may have as few as fifteen pieces/components. Of course, the quality of the fabric, the Lycra, the elastic and lace will be lower. The materials, the design, the hand-cutting and sewing that goes into better bras really does make for higher quality.

"How long should a good bra last?"

While there's no prescribed life for your average bra, it's not uncommon for lace bras to last several years while microfiber/Lycra bras can last up to eighteen months. The way you care for your bra can make all the difference. Don't wear the same bra every day. Rotate your selections. Give your bras time off for good behavior!

"I dearly want to wear a strapless bra, but they never look good on me."

Strapless bras that don't have a formed cup can often collapse, leaving you with breasts that look like two bananas in a sling. Look for a light, contour cup that offers natural cup shape and doesn't compress the upper volume of the breasts.

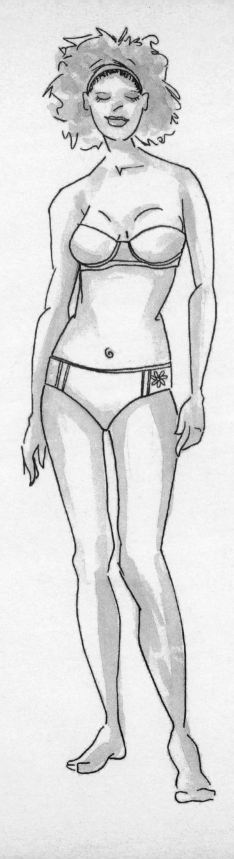

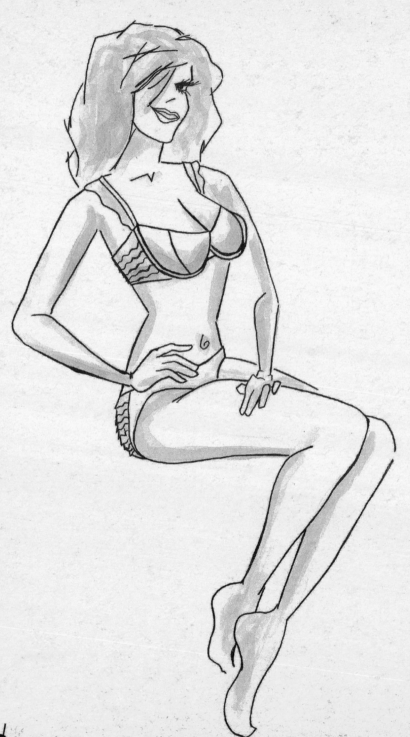

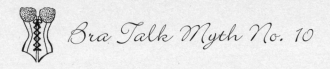

Underwire bras aren't healthy or comfortable.

"My friend, an old hippy, says those bras just aren't natural."

Even the name, *underwire*, sounds horrible. Who in their right mind wants to wear *wires* on their bodies for support? Some women are so philosophically opposed to these u-shaped wires that I have to take two giant steps back before I try to explain why underwire bras are beneficial for support and lift.

If your bra is fitted correctly, you shouldn't notice the underwire. Most are covered with cotton felt, so they feel soft against the chest wall. Plus, they're made of flexible metals with a flat surface that doesn't dig into the skin.

The key to underwire comfort is a firm-fitting bra that doesn't shift on your body, causing the underwire to lose stability. The underwire should lay flat against your rib cage and should not angle upward into the sides or bottom of your breasts. As with most fitting issues, the success of an underwire depends on two factors:

Your Back Band

If the bottom curve of your underwire digs into your chest, it's a sign your bra's back band isn't sufficiently firm. Think of a see-saw. When one side goes down (your falling bust) the other side goes up. To *balance* the see-saw, you've got to have strong legs. Likewise, your bra's back band must be strong enough to stabilize your breasts.

Your Cup Size

A cup that's too small often creates underwire discomfort. You're stressing the cup's ability to contain and lift the bosom. Go one cup size larger, and you'll reduce the tension between the bra and the bust. You'll evenly distribute your breasts' weight in the underwire cup. I always tell women if the bra doesn't fit right it will struggle with the body — and usually the bra wins!

> **Bra Talk** Tip: If you have scar tissue, if you're still healing from recent surgery, or if you're pregnant or nursing, you should consider a soft cup or a soft, ample-fit bra cup.

Doctors are often reluctant to allow breast-implant patients to return to an underwire bra until they've healed and the swelling has gone down, usually about six-to-eight weeks. Some doctors worry that most patients will wear a poorly fitting bra that allows the underwire to press on the healing breast tissue and implant. This is why they recommend a soft cup.

If you're pregnant or nursing, an underwire might interfere with the function of your milk ducts. In your last trimester, and when nursing, consider a soft-cup, seamed bra and a flexible or fuller cup that allows you to grow as the breast tissue swells and releases milk.

Bra Talk **From The Heart**

- Robin's Story -

Dear Susan,

As a forty-something suburban mom, I was getting to the point that I thought I had an unusual or 'abnormal' body. I would shop for bras from store to store, with no luck finding any that were comfortable and looked good as well.

When I arrived for my bra consultation, my fitter guessed my size right there on the spot, before I even undressed. She confirmed the fact that I am full-breasted (which is why all my old bras really never fit right and showed bra lines under my t-shirts, which I *hated*!) She said I should be in a D cup, which shocked me no end, as I am petite, small-boned, and had always worn a B, or maybe, sometimes a C. It turned out that my bras needed alteration. Who would have *ever* thought of having a bra altered? I had just a little taken out here or there, and added some soft material to cover a scratchy section near the hooks in the back.

I began feeling like a new woman — longer, leaner, trimmer, and more proportioned (and more confident!).

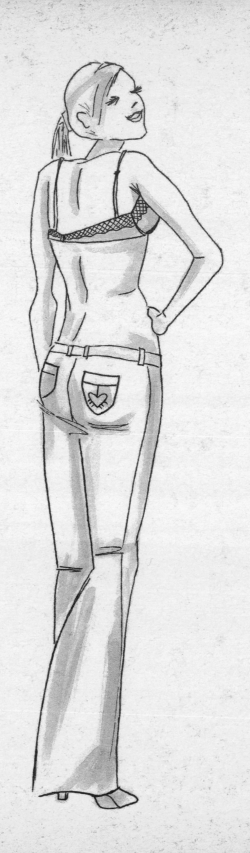

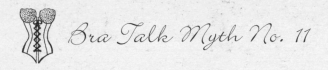

Bulging back fat means the bra's too tight.

"I look like I have 'six-pack abs,' only they're between my shoulder blades. Help!"

Back fat! That's the newest issue to hit the fashion headlines. Everyone's obsessing about the soft tissue that covers our upper backs. Yes, those little bulges are unattractive when you're wearing a conforming t-shirt, but it's not like you're helpless to fight this "battle of the bulge." Call *back fat* your enemy if you like, but I've got the solution.

> **Bra Talk Tip:** Back fat can be almost entirely eliminated if your bra band is positioned lower on your back. If you're fuller-figured, then you may not completely eradicate soft tissue, but the bra band will sit lower on your back, where your shirt is less conforming. Isn't that the most important issue – being a "no show" when you're out and about? When a bra fits well, and your bust is well-lifted, no one will *notice* your back. And if someone *dares* to look under your arm or at your back, then they're *not* your friend. I tell women to disconnect immediately from a relationship with anyone who checks out their back fat! Who needs friends like that?

The proper position of your back band is *level across the narrow part of your back beneath your shoulder blades*. Try it. When you position your back band correctly by pulling it down, your bra will feel more comfortable, it will give you better lift, and your back fat will vanish completely!

"That can't be true," women tell me. "Don't I need a wider back band, instead?"

Nope. You need a *snugger* back band, that's all. When your back band rides up, it pushes your skin and tissue into a bulge. Bulging back fat raises its ugly head even on women who have little or no body fat!

Look at your back in a mirror, and see what I mean. Even when a woman gains weight on other parts of her body, her back remains relatively fat free. Can you imagine the relief when a woman puts on the correct bra and watches the bulge disappear? I promise you, it's not magic — it's just a properly fitted bra!

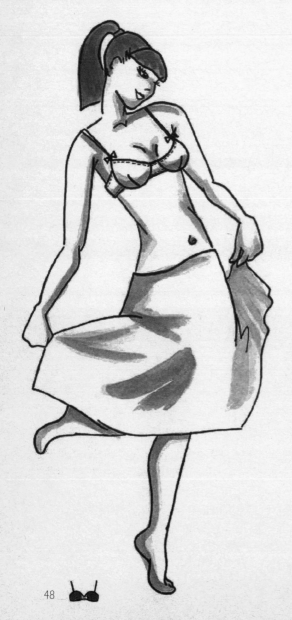

Bra Talk Tips

Shoulder Straps Versus The Back Band

Most women rely on their shoulder straps to hold their bras on their bodies. The bra band rides up a woman's back and can't give her the necessary support because it's too loose. A bra is designed with the band providing enough strength to lift the front bust line. The elastic stretches, and as it retracts it "grabs" or holds the body for 14-16 hours a day. Think how hard your bra works to support you.

The back band must be level with the lowest point on your underwire across the body or even one inch *lower* in the back to provide proper lift. When the back band is level — so that its elastic tension is spread evenly around the body — it can give you the lift you desire. Much like a bridge that needs lateral support (side-to-side,) the structure of a bra must be firmly anchored around the body in order to lift the center over a wide distance.

The straps of the bra should be viewed as stabilizers. They help the bra stay positioned on the body and enable it to adjust for your movements throughout the day — getting in and out of the car, reaching for a coffee cup, bending for a pencil you dropped, and all the other actions you take in your busy and active life.

Only ten percent of a bra's support should come from the straps.

Yet most women rely on the straps. Why?

When your bra band is too loose and the bra rides up your back, your straps fall down. Research shows that over sixty percent of all women complain that their straps fall down throughout the day. Most women believe the problem's caused by their posture and their figures, but this isn't true. Our bodies are just fine!

To correct the problem, women tighten the straps as far as they'll go. Then and only then can the straps actually stay up. But when you shorten your shoulder straps that way, the bra no longer can support your breasts properly.

It becomes a harness! How many of us would feel comfortable wearing a *harness* all day long? It's no wonder women complain about bras being uncomfortable.

So the answer to this dilemma is "Let go." Let go of your shoulder straps. You'll achieve stability in your bra if your back band is level and snug on your body. The weight of your breasts will no longer hang from your shoulders. Imagine the comfort you'll experience and the freedom you'll feel!

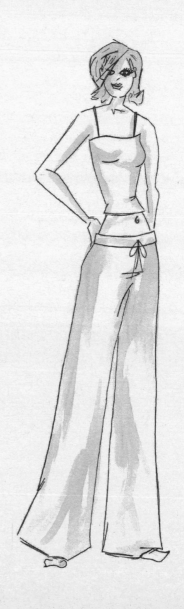

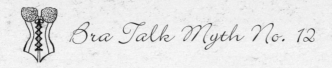
Bra Talk Myth No. 12

Push-up bras give more lift than other bras

"Quick! I just bought a low-cut evening gown, and I need cleavage!"

The rage for push-up bras will always be with us because we all want the look of a firm, high, youthful bust line. "I want cleavage!" is the mantra of fashionable women — especially those in their twenties and thirties. The question is: Are push-up bras all that different from other bras?

Not really. All bras are designed to lift the breasts. Some use plunging cup lines to expose our inner breasts and give our breasts a bit more show, but *all* bras should provide the same lift.

This provokes another question: "So how high should my bust be?"

> **Bra Talk Tip:** Once a woman matures, (mid-twenties and older,) her breasts settle naturally about midway between the tops of her shoulders and her elbows. Take a look at yourself in the mirror (standing sideways, and wearing a bra.) Does your bust fall below that midpoint? If so, it's time for an expert bra fitting and/or a better bra. You'll love this simple test! It'll give you a quick, excellent reference point for determining whether your bra is falling down on the job!

Let's Talk **About Breast Implants**

If you're considering breast implants, do your bra homework, first!

Before you visit any plastic surgeon, have a professional bra fitter size you up so you'll know exactly where you're starting. Ask the fitter to let you try on the next two *deeper* cup sizes with gel inserts (each gel represents one added cup size.)

Do you like the results? Good! Now you have some size guidelines to share with your surgeon. You can even take along the gel insert(s) for show-and-tell. Most doctors are happy to weigh and measure the inserts, then match that size to the implants. That way, you'll get the breast size you like.

Don't assume your surgeon will understand your expectations, otherwise. I've talked to a lot of plastic surgeons about breast issues, and I guarantee you, most don't know diddly about bra cup sizes. They only know how to describe breasts in terms like "volume of liquid!"

Without clear guidance from you, most surgeons will make your breasts larger than you expected. Immediately after surgery your breasts will be swollen, so it may be weeks before you realize how big they are. Then it's too late to change your mind.

In my experience, many women who have breast enhancement surgery are surprised and disappointed when they discover all those gorgeous bras they planned to wear don't work well for their new, larger cup size.

And keep this in mind, too: If you gain weight later, as many women do, your enhanced bust will get even larger. So take charge, ask the right questions, and tell your surgeon exactly what you want! It's your body. Be clear from the start!

> **Bra Talk Tip:** Bras that clasp in the front are sleek in appearance and easy to slip on – or off! — but they last only a third as long as the average back-clasp bra. Why? They generally have only one hook to clasp, so the bra band quickly loses firmness and begins to shift when you move.

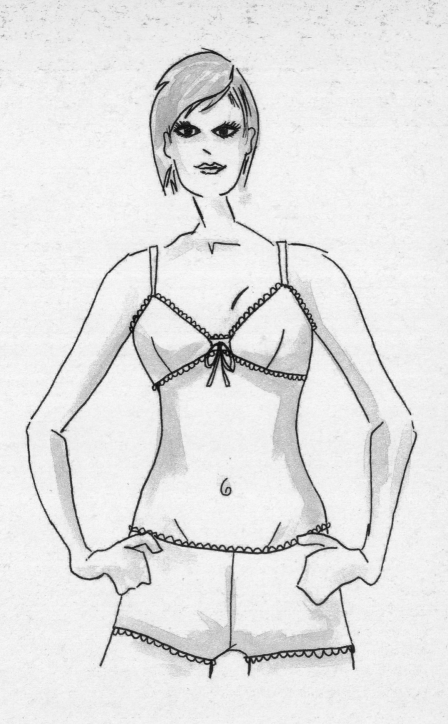

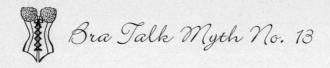 *Bra Talk Myth No. 13*

Exercise can firm breast tissue

"I work out like an Olympic weight lifter.
Why don't my breasts look better?"

Don't we wish!

When you exercise, you're working the pectoral muscles that lay over your rib cage and under your breasts. Since the pectorals support your breast tissue, yes, if you tone them up, your breasts may look a little higher.

Unfortunately, for most of us, the effect is minimal. You'll have to pump a tremendous amount of iron to create a significant change in your appearance, and it won't improve the firmness of the breast itself, since the breast tissue is not muscle.

The truth is, our breasts are composed of milk glands, fat and other fibrous tissues. Each breast is given its shape by membranes called *Cooper's Ligaments*. Without the support of a good bra, these cone-shaped ligaments will stretch and lose their elasticity, resulting in permanent sagging.

Bra Talk Tip: Elasticity cannot be regained once the ligaments are stretched. Wearing a bra prevents this loss of firmness. If you exercise without wearing a proper sports bra, you may cause breast injury and tenderness. For many, the damage is irreversible! Only surgical reconstruction of the breast can restore their shape and a more youthful appearance.

Bra Talk Tip: Keep a mixture of bras in your wardrobe. Is it a hot summer day? Forget your padded cups and go seamless in a sexy, sheer bra. Feeling frilly? Wear lace to make you feel feminine and boob-a-licious!

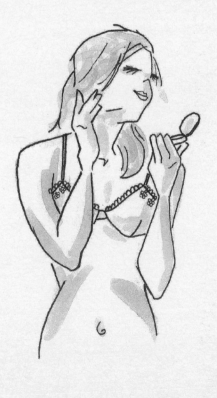

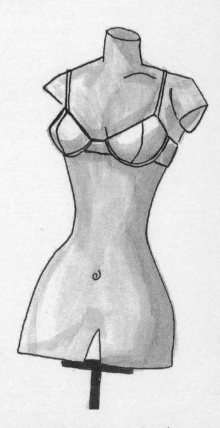

Bra Talk **From The Heart**

- Leyla's Story -

Dear Susan,

I was wearing a 38DD and was constantly uncomfortable. My bra never fully covered my breasts and it was always digging into my ribs no matter how tightly I adjusted the straps. I always dreaded the trip to the department store to buy a new bra because not only did they never have one that would fit, but also, the largest ones they had were in the least attractive styles.

It was not until my first trip to *Intimacy* that I was able to finally purchase 'fun' bras. It turns out that I am really a 32G. The first time I tried on a bra in that size I could immediately feel and see the difference.

No longer was the bra digging into my ribs, and I also looked as if I had lost ten pounds! It made me feel more confident and comfortable. I no longer had to push my bra up every few hours.

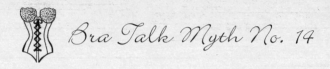

Bra Talk Myth No. 14

Only padded bras can hide happy nipples.

"I'm all for the natural look, but I turn three shades of purple when there's show-through."

We're understandably concerned with exposing ourselves in front of co-workers, family members or at Great Aunt Nona's funeral. It's a little horrifying to find that your headlights are showing for all to see. In general, women are modest and want to prevent a public display.

With proper positioning of the breast in the center of the cup, and with a stable underwire as back-up, most nipple misbehavior can be eliminated. Nipples react to irritation. They're sensitive to the shifting movements of your bra's fabric. But if you position your nipple on the center seam, it masks show-through and prevents those embarrassing personal moments. The cup seam is the strongest stress point in your bra's design. It can control a wayward nipple!

If you feel you still have "show-and-tell nipples," try a lightly-lined contour bra or a double-lined fabric in a seamless, molded cup. Either will mask any nipple hi-jinks. The contour bras also add shape and create a smooth surface for your casual t-shirts and knit tops.

As a last resort, you can stick Band-Aids over your nipples. I recommend the ones made of non-woven material in decorative flower or circular shapes. Have some fun!

> **Bra Talk Tip:** Instead of standard Band-Aid-like cover-ups, try the newest gel cover-ups, such as *Dimmers* and *Bra Disks*. They're contoured on the edges. You'll get a smoother look.

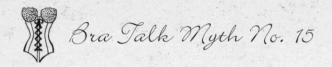

Sport bras are supposed to fit and look like a sweaty tube sock.

> "I hate wearing the 'uni-boob style' when I exercise.
> Are there alternatives?"

Whether you're running in the Olympics or just racing down the aisles of your grocery store, active lifestyles require *proactive* support. A good sports bra is a necessity!

A sports bra reduces the strain and impact caused by extreme breast movement. Many women are embarrassed to discuss the subject of their bouncing bust line, yet the truth is, inadequate breast support causes sore and tender breasts that can derail your exercise regimen.

You think pulled calf muscles and aching knee joints are bad?

According to Dr. Julia Alleyne, Medical Director, Sports Medicine, University of Toronto and Sunnybrook-Women's College Hospital, here are just a few of the miseries the wrong sports bra can inflict on your jiggling bosom:

Chafing, bruising, abrasions, something sinister-sounding called *breast displacement*, and general skin irritation, due to trapped sweat.

Ouch!

Some women try to outsmart their breasts by doubling up on the popular, crop-top *compression* sports bras — you know, the cotton Lycra bandeaus that mash your breasts to your chest wall. But compression-type sports bras encourage your breasts to move as a solid block.

You now have a uni-boob.

Not only is the *uni-boob* unattractive, it *definitely* won't give you the best support. Lack of support means you bounce too much, straining the base root tissue of your breasts, which can be painful.

Bra Talk Tip: Buy a sports bra that offers you cup-shaped, *seamed* support. Stitched seams provide strength along with support, evenly distributing motion stresses across the entire breast. Seamed cups can even be designed to accommodate the stresses of specific sports – such as tennis or golf — with vertical seams for side-to-side movement. Also look for moisture-wicking properties in the bra's fabric, to prevent chafing and other skin irritations.

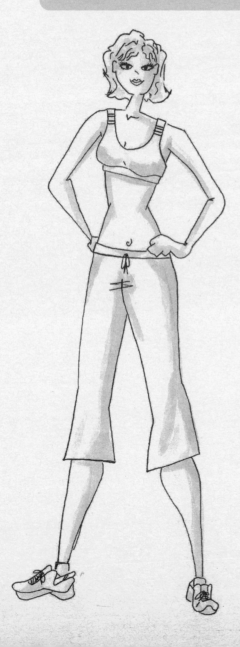

This typical "crop top" doesn't provide support.

Dear Bra Talk: My mom used to say, 'It's better to have too much than not enough.'

Bra Talk Tips For Teens

As a pre-teen or young-teen girl approaches puberty, she'll likely find her breasts are more developed than her mother's were at that age and that she menstruates much earlier than her mother's generation did. It's true that each generation of young women is maturing earlier and are more "busty" than the previous. I'm betting that each successive generation of women will be at least one cup size larger. Why is that so?

Researchers say the culprit could easily be our modern diet. We eat more, including high-fat fast foods. Plus we're ingesting hormones from our food processes that have an effect on the size and weight of young women.

Today, a full D cup is pretty average for a young adult woman. Since most women are very size conscious, this may come as a unwelcome surprise! Take heart: Don't be overly concerned with the labeling of your cup size. Just strive to get the right fit for your bra. You'll look fine.

During ages 13-to-18, a girl should be fitted for a bra at least once a year. With hormonal changes and an active lifestyle (sports, parties, diet) it's likely she'll need increasing support. Some teens go through growth spurts. Some may need a new cup size to accommodate their changing teen fashions and to fit in with their peer group.

This is a challenging time for most girls, and they're now *super* self-conscious about their changing bodies! Weight changes and the associated stretch marks can easily damage a teen's confidence.

Whether she's an outgoing gal who's leading the social pack or she's a late bloomer, she's thinking about her evolving shape all the time. She's often concerned with her weight, bust line or just what style and dress are acceptable. You can help your daughter feel her best during these changes by helping her get the right bra in terms of support and also individual style.

Bra Talk Tip: To make your breasts look plumper, bend over while you put on your bra. Center your nipples above the mid-point in the cups to get top volume. To show off your cleavage, select a *demi-plunge bra* or a *contour-plunge bra.* Both create fullness in the center of your breasts.

Bra Talk Tip: Do you want your breasts to have a rounder shape? Then choose a bra with *seamless* cups. Seamless bras generally create a more natural appearance than seamed cups (when fit properly.) Just remember: Seamless cups generally have less depth than seamed cups, so you may have to go up one cup size. Try it and see what happens!

Bra Talk **From The Heart**

- *Karen's Story* -

Dear Susan,

This past year, at thirty-seven, I was diagnosed with breast cancer. When my doctor said it was okay for me to wear a bra again (after reconstructive surgery) I wasn't sure what to buy. I had never worn a bra without an underwire, not to mention that my entire body had changed shape, so I was unclear as to my cup size. My first call (walking in *bald*,) was to your store.

Your staff greeted me with love and respect. The experience of having a real bra fitting is hard to put into words.

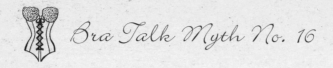 *Bra Talk Myth No. 16*

It's impossible to pick out a good bra without an expert's help.

"Okay, I don't have a personal bra coach. What should I do?"

You're standing alone in the claustrophobic dressing room of Giganto Department Store. In your hand is a bra you plucked off the racks in the lingerie department. You're wondering if it's the perfect bra for you, or just another disappointing Zombie Bra of Doom.

"If only a professional bra fitter were here to advise me!" you whisper nervously.

Relax! There are easy ways to tell whether a bra will give you the performance your life and body demand. This three-step process will help you pick the best cup size, the best shape and the most comfortable fit:

1. Fasten the bra's back band, position the cups under your breasts, and bend to your waist. Let your breasts fall gently into the cups. This automatically centers your breasts in the cups and assures even weight distribution. Don't lift or grab your breasts and pull them into the cups. Be gentle. Your body appreciates the same soft touch you might use in applying skin moisturizer to your face.

2. Ease the bra into place, make sure the back band is centered, and lift the straps onto your shoulders. Your breasts shouldn't bulge out of the cups. Your nipples should be centered in the cups, and the tops of your breasts should look nice and full.

3. Release the fabric on the tops of the cups to help your breasts settle even better. Insert your forefinger at the center of each cup and slide it to the side of the cup. Use your forefinger like a spatula to adjust your breasts. This smoothes the breast, eliminating any wrinkles or puckering of the cup or your skin.

If the cup is too shallow, then go down a cup size. If the cup is too full, go up a cup size. When you raise your arms, see if the bra moves with you. You don't want it to lift or shift when it's brand new!

Looks good? Wonderful! See, you can do it!

> **Bra Talk Tip:** If you're like most women, one of your breasts is slightly larger than the other. When you're fitted for a bra, always fit the fuller breast first. If the cup wrinkles on the smaller side, you can custom-alter the bra's back on that (smaller) side. Generally, that means pulling the underwire back one-half to one inch, for a personalized fit.

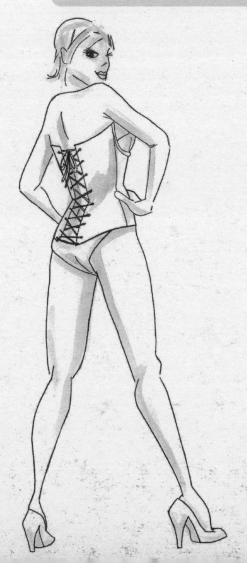

Bra Talk **From The Heart**

- Tanya's Story -

Dear Susan,

After having lost 133 pounds, I have a lot of excess skin. I have searched high
and low for a bra that would help. Every bra I tried did not give me enough
support or lift. When I went to your shop, your sales clerk was able to just look
at me and bring back the exact size I needed.

All self-consciousness is gone. I am able to wear tight-fitting blouses and my
breasts look right. I look like I've had breast surgery! Thank you so much!

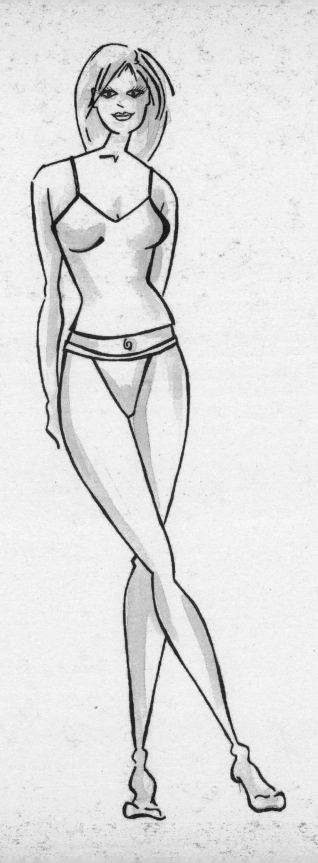

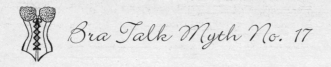 *Bra Talk Myth No. 17*

Picking a bra is a science, not an art

"How come you don't believe in tape measures?
That's un-American!"

I believe in a holistic method of bra fitting that personalizes the bra fitting process to your body and does not involve a tape measure. Most experienced fitters can tell what size a woman is — or estimate closely — by sight alone. Remember, fitting a bra is a very individual process, and each bra may fit a little differently depending upon its style and size. This is why fitting specialists use their knowledge and experience to help clients decide which bras are best.

The traditional tape measure method involves measuring under the bust and then over the bust, followed by calculations to give a cup size recommendation. Fair enough. But *where* you measure on the body is the most problematic issue. If you measure one inch higher on a woman's back, her circumference (body width) will be dramatically different.

This is why the tape measure method is so often incorrect or misleading. I've been measured by various stores, with conflicting results no less than *five* times. Do you wonder why I distrust this technique?

Fitting a bra isn't an exact science, even though some retailers and bra manufacturers seem to think so! While measuring seems to provide quantitative answers, if often falls apart when the bras are tested in the dressing room. The materials, the company size standards, and the cup type will ultimately determine the stretch and width of the bra.

> **Bra Talk Tip:** You've always heard that bras should "lift and separate," right? But if you want to look your best, buy bras that separate your breasts *only one inch — or less!* Don't spread your girlfriends across different time zones!

Bra Talk Tip: Think you can't wear a strapless bra? Plagued by fears of a fatal, falling, fashion *faux pas?* Just go *down* one size in your back band and *up* two sizes in your cups. The bigger cups won't look funny, I promise, because, generally, strapless cups are more shallow than your regular cups. Strapless bras fall down for one simple reason: a loose back band. By combining a tighter band and fuller cup you'll get the support and stability you need. Dance that tango!

Bra Talk **From The Heart**

Dear Susan,

I am an actor, singer and dancer. I love what I do. I love telling stories through my body — creating fleeting, ephemeral works of art, such as the nature of life. Unfortunately, in recent years I have felt my body begin to rebel against me. I had always had *boundless* energy, and because of all the dancing I do, in class or recreationally I am quite strong.

However, despite going to the gym, running, and dancing, my breasts have continued to get bigger. My clothes kept fitting more and more poorly. I was wearing at least *two* bras to go to the gym or out running, and whenever I caught a glimpse of myself walking down the street, I was horrified at how disproportionate I looked.

And I felt it, too.

I cannot express how strange it feels to have these *things* on your chest bounding around! Everyone looks at you, and you feel it has nothing to do with you or what you're about. One of my fondest memories was quickly becoming when I got to play the Artful Dodger for in a production of *Oliver Twist*. The show allowed me to bind myself, because I was playing a boy. Ah, the freedom!

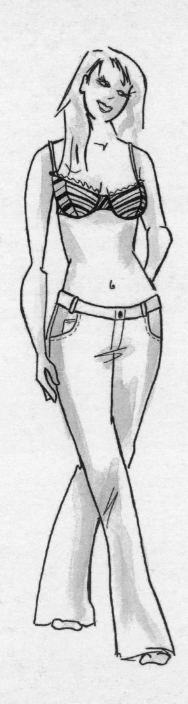

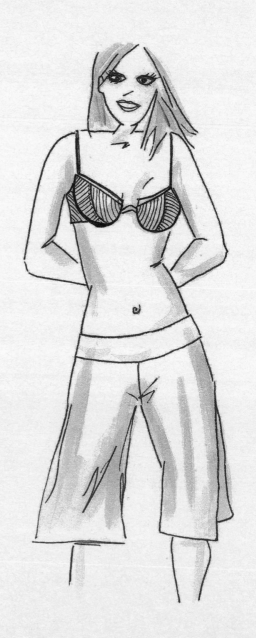

"Men can be cruel and lewd."

I called my parents in hysterics a couple of times. I wanted breast reduction surgery. Of course, being a performing artist, I could not even *dream* of being able to pay for that on my own. Even getting more work and pay than most of my fellow performers, it is still laughable how much artists must work at other jobs just to make the rent and scrape by on the bills.

Yet I felt I had no choice if I wanted keep up with my exercise routines or look good in my dance theater company. I was uncomfortable and miserable in my body and in my heart.

Men can be cruel and lewd, and never let me forget a second what I looked like. And I, about a 34D but on a petite and relatively delicate but strong frame, felt like a *freak*.

My parents began looking at doctors, and I investigated whether any kind of health insurance would cover this kind of operation (probably not.) I was dead set on getting it done soon.

"I was flabbergasted."

Then my mom watched an episode of *The Oprah Winfrey Show*, in which you and your advice were featured. Mom was *amazed* at the differences in the women's appearances after they changed bras, and noted that some of them were much larger sizes than me. She phoned immediately and told me to go as soon as I could to your store, so that — at least until I had surgery — some new, special bras could provide a temporary solution.

I am still surprised as can be that your store provided a permanent solution. The sales girl who waited on me — exactly my age at 24 — was jovial and so helpful. She put me immediately at ease, and showed me, in what seemed like only thirty glorious seconds, about ten bras that seemed to reduce my breast size by at least one cup. I was flabbergasted. She had answers to every question that I asked.

"I'm happy and healthy again."

When I checked out of the store with three new regular bras, and one new sports bra for dance and running, the girls at the cash register applauded and said they would come see me perform when I was famous. They were all thrilled for my rediscovered comfort in my body, which is, as we say, my instrument.

I'm back out running and dancing, and even though I am still a *busty* girl, as the guys on the street might say, I don't feel like a victim of the way I was made, anymore. So those guys can't make me feel like one, either. And there are no scalpels anywhere in sight! Thank you, so much. And my parents thank you, too, for making their little girl happy and healthy again. And for obliterating a very, *very* large medical bill.

Letter from a Bra

Dear Sally,

We've been breast friends for so long! I've remained your bosom buddy through thick and thin. I've tried so hard to lift you up and satisfy all your needs. But now — we're not supporting one another. Let's face the truth:

I'm falling down all the time.
I cause you pain whenever I'm near you.
I'm not as supportive as I used to be.

You need someone new to lift your body and spirits. So please, get the help you need to re-awaken your real beauty. I hope you'll find a new soul mate and chest buddy.

Goodbye forever,

Your Old Bra

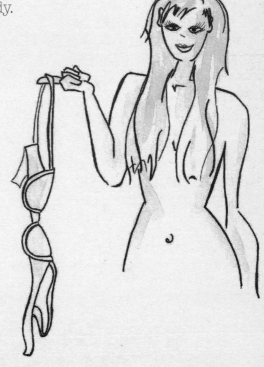

A Note From Susan Nethero

- Her Own Story -

All throughout this book I've talked about the most personal feelings and confessions that women have shared with me. Now it's time for me to tell you my story.

Why am I so passionate about bust lines and bras?

As a late bloomer, I struggled to find fashionable styles that made me feel special. When my mom took me to our local lingerie store, I would just cringe! I remember the disappointment I felt when that little gray-haired sales lady would suggest a soft-cup bra on a lacy camisole. Didn't she *get* it? All I wanted was definition and a lacy bra! And then there were the trends.

Do you remember "Twiggy" in the 1960's? She was my idol, short-haired and flat-chested! Or how about the seventies? When *everybody* went braless. (Do you remember burning bras as a symbol of the fight against the "Establishment?") Those trends didn't last long enough for *me*.

During my twenties, I learned I could get great bras in my size (a perfect fit) in Europe. European designers, who make a wide range of sizes, from A to JJ cups, are unparalleled in their devotion to quality, style and fashion for every woman. All through my business career I was concerned about getting professional attire that would fit my small bust and full hips.

That's when I discovered *gel inserts* that would fit in any bra. Nope, I never considered breast enhancement! It just seemed unnatural for me. But I loved the gel inserts, and I still wear them today (in various sizes, depending on how full-busted I want to be.)

Today, changing my cup size is like getting a new haircut or makeover — I do it for *me*.

After I spent nearly twenty years working in senior executive and marketing assignments for the corporate business world — employed by giants like *Dow*, *Xerox*, and *Time, Inc.*, I decided to start my own venture as a "bra fit specialty retailer." *Intimacy Bra Fitting Specialists* was born in 1992. This journey began with world-renowned British bra-fitting guru June Kenton — the official bra fitter to Queen Elizabeth — who taught me all about fitting and product design.

June didn't realize that American women were still in the dark ages when it came to professional bra-fitting advice. At the time, no one was providing that service for women in the United States. Well, fourteen years later, I can honestly say we've changed the situation! At *Intimacy Bra Fitting Specialists* we've personally fit over 500,000 women in our stores!

Almost every customer we serve tells us life-changing stories about her improved comfort and fit, not to mention the emotional benefits to her lifestyle. The gratitude of our customers inspires our fitting consultants daily. Our corporate philosophy is simple:

We want to empower and uplift women.

That is the *Intimacy* way.

We eat, drink and live for the opportunity to help women look better and feel better. Our careers have become our life purpose, and our employees and our customers are our dearest friends.

Happy Fittings!

Susan

All About
Intimacy Bra Fitting Specialists

At *Intimacy, Bra Fitting Specialists*, our aim is to enhance a woman's sense of inner beauty through her most intimate foundations. We are committed to serving the fit, comfort and definition needs of women of all shapes and sizes, providing fashionable lingerie from the international market.

Whether you are a tailored businesswoman or a "girly girl," we offer you a wide selection from the best designers around the world. Our selection is rich with basics for a casual lifestyle but also wickedly *fun* for the woman with a playful fashion appetite.

We actively search the market for unique — but also *proven* — bras in an extraordinary range of shapes, designs, quality, and sizes. We pride ourselves on a selection that offers something for women from the petite A cup to the full JJ cup, in band widths from 30 to 44 inches.

We've always got an eye out for new styles and fashions for every cup size, from the strapless, "demi-est" of fashions to the practical sport, nursing and even *sleeping* bras — yes, that's right, *Intimacy* carries bras designed specifically for bedtime wear. Our sleeping bras are a great selection for fuller-busted women or for those who want extra comfort for those special times when their breasts are tender.

No hassles, no embarrassment

At *Intimacy*, our fitters are experienced style and fit *gurus*! They're both passionate and *compassionate* about *uplifting* women at all stages of life. We train them in the *Intimacy* holistic bra-fit process so they can help every woman achieve the comfort, fit, and shape she desires.

You don't ever have to worry about feeling shy or embarrassed when you come in for a fitting at one of our shops. We take utmost care to protect your privacy and to honor your feelings. Don't forget — I was a victim of an insensitive bra fitter when I was a young woman — and so, I promise we will give *you* all the respect and attention you deserve.

We're all about "can do," and we won't dismiss your special desires — we may, however, gently tell you the *truth*, if a particular style doesn't compliment your shape or gives you marginal fit and look. You deserve our expert advice, and that includes our honesty. But we promise you'll leave our shops feeling new inner confidence, thanks to the proper bra fit and styling for your busy life!

"*Intimacy* improved the way I look on the outside and the way I feel on the inside! I had no idea I'd been wearing the wrong size bra all these years until *Intimacy* fitted me to my *true* size. The benefits are unbelievable. I'm so much more comfortable. I feel like a whole new woman!"

That's a story we hear all the time at our shops. We welcome you today for a personalized bra fitting!

About our locations

Intimacy opened its flagship store in 1992 at fashionable Phipps Plaza, Atlanta's premiere upscale mall. In 2004, we acquired *Roberta's*, a well-known lingerie boutique on Madison Avenue in New York, so we could bring our bra fitting expertise, our wide selection and our *Intimacy* reputation for customer service to the Big Apple.

This fall we will open our *third* store, on Chicago's fabulous "Miracle Mile," at 900 North Michigan. We're so excited about this opportunity to bring our *enhancing* women's lingerie, our fabulous fit and fashion, to the midwest.

We're proud to say that last year *Intimacy Bra Fitting Specialists* was named "Best Reference Shop in North America" at an international exposition hosted by *Intima* magazine. You'll see how we earned that honor when you visit our shops in Atlanta, New York, and Chicago. We look forward to fitting you with the bras of your dreams!

Join us on our website for the latest, greatest bra-fit tips and techniques

Our *Intimacy* website, at *www.myintimacy.com*, is designed to give women easy access to a world of bra tips, myths, facts, style and fashion.

The site will provide you with helpful information about the brands and sizes we carry, but you'll also enjoy these great features:

- The Top Ten Bra Myths
- Most Frequently Asked Questions About Bras

- "What's My Size," an interactive module that will help you determine *your size!*
- "Store Locator," a resource for women to find a bra-fitting store in their area. To date, we list over 100 stores in thirty-two states! There are bra-fitting specialty stores throughout the USA!

We plan to make www.myintimacy.com the electronic world's leading site for bra-fitting information!

Coming soon:

- "Before and After"
- "Anatomy of Breast Tissue"
- "How to Put On A Bra" with June Kenton from *Rigby & Peller* — the famous British bra designer and personal fitter for Queen Elizabeth!

Last but not least, we invite you to sign up for our "e-blasts" — the latest info on bra-fitting advances, special news coverage, promotional offers, and much more! Our monthly newsletter promises to be your very best resource for bra-fitting information.

See you soon!

Susan

Your Bra Talk Check List

How to analyze your bra needs

If you have experienced any of the following challenges with bra feelings please visit your nearest Intimacy boutique or a bra fitting specialty store. To find a store location near you see www.myintimacy.com.

Do you ever have problems with the following?

- ❏ Bra straps falling down
- ❏ Need more bust volume
- ❏ Need or want more support — not as firm as used to be
- ❏ Underwire digging into breast tissue
- ❏ Straps dig into shoulder
- ❏ One breast larger than other
- ❏ Back of bra (band) rides up back
- ❏ Appearance of back fat
- ❏ Breast tissue comes out underneath the underwire
- ❏ Soft breast tissue—pendulous breast

Have you experienced any of the following life changes

- ❏ Increase in exercise
- ❏ Pregnancy or childbirth
- ❏ Nursing
- ❏ Weight loss
- ❏ Enhancements or breast reduction
- ❏ Birth control or menopause medications

Your Bra Talk Personal Diary

Use these pages to record your bra history for easy reference.

Date: _____

My Bra's Brand Name: _____

Bra Style: _____

Store Where Purchased: _____

Cup Size: _____

Band Width: _____

Special Features: _____
_____

My Current Needs: _____
_____
_____
_____

Other Notes: _____
_____
_____
_____

Date: _____

My Bra's Brand Name: _____

Bra Style: _____

Store Where Purchased: _____

Cup Size: _____

Band Width: _____

Special Features: _____
_____

My Current Needs: _____
_____
_____

Other Notes: _____
_____
_____
_____

Date: _____

My Bra's Brand Name: _____

Bra Style: _____

Store Where Purchased: _____

Cup Size: _____

Band Width: _____

Special Features: _____

_____

My Current Needs: _____

_____

_____

_____

Other Notes: _____

_____

_____

_____

_____

Date: _____

My Bra's Brand Name: _____

Bra Style: _____

Store Where Purchased: _____

Cup Size: _____

Band Width: _____

Special Features: _____

_____

My Current Needs: _____

_____

_____

_____

Other Notes: _____

_____

_____

_____

At **INTIMACY** and other bra and specialty stores, your records are protected for your privacy and kept on file for your convenience.

Where To Find Bra Talk

Bra Talk is available at all locations of *Intimacy Bra Fitting Specialists* and, for those who prefer the e-commerce world of on-line shopping, at www.myintimacy.com.

Atlanta: Phipps Plaza, Atlanta, GA , (404) 261-9333

New York: 1252 Madison Avenue (Corner of 90th and Madison) New York, NY, (212) 860-8366

Chicago: 900 Michigan Avenue, (3rd Floor), Chicago, IL

Visit *Intimacy* and Susan Nethero at www.MyIntimacy.com
   or call us at 1(877) A2HHCUP

Bra Talk is also available at fine bookstores everywhere, and direct from BelleBooks.

BelleBooks
Good Books. Fine People.
P.O. Box 67 , Smyrna, GA 30081
(770) 384-1348
bellebooks@bellebooks.com

Booksellers and librarians: BelleBooks titles can be ordered through these major wholesalers: Ingram, Baker & Taylor, and Brodart.

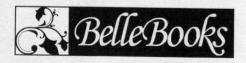

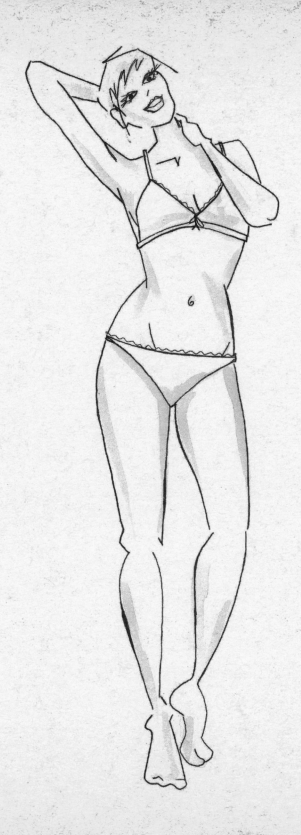

Bra Talk with Susan Nethero
In The News

Great articles and TV appearances featuring more of Susan's advice.

New York Daily News	January 2005
Parenting Magazine	March 2005
Marie Claire Magazine	April 2005
Life and Style Magazine	April 2005
The Oprah Winfrey Show	May 20, 2005
www2.oprah.com/tows/pastshows/ 200505/tows_past_20050520_c.jhtml	
O Magazine	July 2005
www.oprah.com/omagazine/200507/omag_200507_bra.jhtml	
New York Post	July 25, 2005
Redbook Magazine	August 2005
Women's Day	August 2005
Parents Magazine	October 2005
Elle Magazine	October 2005

**For Susan's current appearances
and book signing schedules,
see www.myintimacy.com.**

The Mossy Creek Hometown Series

Come home to Mossy Creek. Mitford meets Mayberry in this small north Georgia town filled with eccentrics who share their tales of heartbreak and renewal. These collective novels blend the storytelling talent of a number of authors.

Mossy Creek ❖ Reunion in Mossy Creek ❖ Summer at Mossy Creek
Blessings of Mossy Creek

Coming in Fall 2005

A Day in Mossy Creek

THE SWEET TEA STORY COLLECTIONS

Come sit on the porch a spell. Let's talk about times gone by and folks we remember, about slow summer evenings and lightning bugs in a jar. Let's talk about our wonderful South, both then and now. Short stories by a variety of Southern authors.

Sweet Tea and Jesus Shoes

MORE SWEET TEA

The WaterLilies Series
Southern. Sexy. Mermaids. The ocean is filled with mysteries, and so is the heart. Join New York Times' bestselling author Deborah Smith on a whimsical journey through the supernatural world of a glamourous coastal-Georgia family who have a bit more than the ordinary family secrets to hide.

Alice At Heart

DIARY OF A RADICAL MERMAID

The Everyone's Special Series

Kasey Belle, the Tiniest Fairy in the Kingdom

Kasey Belle is sad to be the tiniest fairy in the magnolia forest until she meets a friendly dragonfly named Rhett and together they win the heart of a fierce giant. An illustrated children's book by veteran author Sandra Chastain and the debut of illustrator Cindy Chadwick.

Astronaut Noodle and The Planet Velocity

Intrepid space explorer Astronaut Noodle sets out to capture the fast-moving citizens of Planet Velocity with his trusty camera. An illustrated children's book. Coming in Fall 2005

BelleBooks Presents Warm-Hearted Novels Of The Heart

All God's Creatures

In 1960, Memphis debutante Maggie McClaine gives up her society crown to become a veterinarian. Follow Dr. McClaine through four decades of life, love, joy, sorrow, and four-footed friends. By veteran author and horsewoman Carolyn McSparren.

Coming in Spring 2006

Creola's Moonbeam

Suffering a mid-life crisis, Atlanta novelist Honey Newberry escapes to the Gulf beaches of Florida. Amidst poignant memories of the wise black woman who raised her, Honey struggles to reclaim her spirit and once again become "Creola's Moonbeam." A BelleBooks' debut by Milam McGraw Propst, Georgia Author of the Year and author of the acclaimed novel The Adventures of Ociee Nash, recently released as a feature film starring Keith Carradine and Mare Winningham.

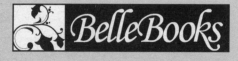

Good Books. Fine People.
(770) 384-1348
P.O. Box 67
Smyrna, GA 30081
BelleBooks@BelleBooks.com
www.bellebooks.com